First Printing July 2018
Copyright © 2018 by Barbara J. Wright
All Rights Reserved.

Cover Design : Pizap
Editor/Publisher: Bernadette Watkins
ISBN: 978-1-387-96862-6

Author's Notes :

AN INVITATION TO HEALTH CARE:
The content of this pamphlet is realized and developed because of my personal journey in association with people during my nursing career. And, experiences with people helped in the creation of a truly authentic pamphlet.

"Prescription for optimum health is knowledge".
This information is not a substitute for healthcare professional advice. I am proud to offer this information to people everywhere. Some information is quotes from, "BOTTOM LINES ULTIMATE HEALING"; (volume 11).

My nursing history motivated me to try and help people to manage their own health to a certain extent. (keep it simple). As a retired nurse, I have the need to be needed syndrome. My Spirit revealed to me that I could help people through writing.

Contact:
barbarajean217@gmail.com

"An Invitation To Health Care"
by Barbara Jean Wright

BIOGRAPHY:
I am a black female age 82 and my former education
includes being a graduate of high school in 1954 and
graduate of college in 1975 and Nursing in 1977 L.P.N./R.N.

Work Experience:
Nurse Aide; Dental Assistant; Nurse; Nutrition Educator;
Geriatric Caregiver Educator;

VOLUNTEER:
Parkinson's Group; Hospice Care.

Community Actives:
President of Church Board; Served on Mental Health
Board; Served on Circle of Care for Families; Served on
Enterprise Community Board.
(current).

HEALTH CARE SELF HELP THROUGH INFORMATION AND EDUCATION:

Options in managing our health; (health care essentials)...

What nurses know and doctors don't tell you... Medical doctors are trained to treat illness; injury; and disease with medication, surgery and hospitalization. They really don't have the time to give detailed self care advice. Nurses are usually the best people to give this advice in order to help patients avoid dangerous mistakes.

WHAT DOCTOR'S SHOULD ASK BUT WON"T:

... about your nutrition; stress levels; personal life; genetic risk factors; *(Also, you must share information and ask questions.)* Remember this is your life.

CONDITIONS DOCTOR'S SOMETIME MISDIAGNOSE:

gastroenteritis;
migraine;
muscle strain;
pleurisy;
 rash;

Ask the doctor if blood work or any test are needed to authenticate the diagnosis.

BEFORE HAVING MINOR SURGERY:
Studies show that it is risky to have surgery in a doctor's office. Consider a surgical center. Get information about surgical procedures. You can do research online about these procedures or ask your local surgical center.

AVOID UNNECESSARY SURGERY:
prostate;
cataract;
wisdom teeth extraction;
gallbladder;

(A second opinion is wise).

FULL BODY SCAN:

A full body scan is questionable. However the medical community recommends people over 40 get a full body scan as a preventive measure. (*Early detection is the best protection*).Today of course, full body scans are common in the medical community. Nevertheless, there are some downsides to full body scans. The one I would be most concerned about is radiation exposure. It has been noted that full body scanning has 10 times more radiation than standard x-rays. Sometimes a followup may be necessary. In some cases insurance doesn't cover it. Also, exposure to radiation is a known risk for cancer.

HOSPITAL HIDDEN KILLER:

Blood clots sometimes don't have symptoms.
However, there are some risk factors:
obesity;
heart failure;
infections;
lung problems;
prolonged
immobility;

When a blood clot forms in the leg and blocks the flow of blood, it can lead to sudden death. If a clot breaks and travels upward through the body and lodges in the lungs. It can cause sudden death. Anyone admitted to a hospital with two or more risk factors must be evaluated and treated appropriately.

HOW TO CHOOSE THE RIGHT HOSPITAL FOR YOUR CONDITION:

There are two major categories of hospitals: general hospitals and specialty hospitals. Specialty hospitals focus on one type of medical condition. General hospital's deal with a variety of medical conditions. In general, people view hospitals as a safe place while they are ill.

According to Health Grades *(a leading healthcare rating company)* 95,000 patients die in hospitals yearly, due to medical errors. However, you have some options. Keep a list of prescribed medications.

Misuse of medications or taking the wrong medications are the most common and dangerous medical errors. Make sure your arm band is checked before taking medications or participating in any other procedure. If you are being operated on mark the area before going to the operating room. If you are too ill to do these things for yourself, ask a family member who can do them for you.

EVERY DAY AILMENTS:

Here's an overview of some of our basic needs for daily living. I believe our Spiritual need is the foundation for all of our needs.

Natural ways to guard against colds, flu, and worse:

***Washing* hands.**
Keeping our hands clean is one of the most important steps we can take. To avoid getting sick, and spreading germs to others, wash your hands often with soap and clean running water.

Nutrition:

"A Lifetime of Wellness"; Diane Hale's 7th edition book , convinced me that we are what we eat. Good nutrition is our lifeline. It affects all of our body organs in an amazing way. We have the USDA food guide pyramid for guidance on eating healthy meals. Proper nutrition will enhance our body, mind, and spirit.

Exercise:

WHAT EXERCISE CAN DO FOR YOU:

It will increase your respiratory capacity and improves digestion.

It strengthens bones, increases joint mobility, and improves your circulation.

It improves your mood, stimulates your brain and reduces your risk of heart disease.

It increases your muscle strength and muscle tone.

CONCLUSION:

I thank God for blessing me with the wisdom and knowledge to hopefully help people understand that they have options regarding managing their health and wellness.

I thank my spouse, children, and grandchildren for their confidence, encouragement, and support.

Author

Personal Notes:

www.ingramcontent.com/pod-product-compliance
Lightning Source LLC
Chambersburg PA
CBHW050354290526
45785CB00006B/2772